Presented to:

Never Forget the
Difference You've Made